CONTENTS

INTRODUCTION

If you're having a problem with chronic inflammation, you'll love this book. It can help to improve your life, and give you the recipes to start this lifestyle change on the right foot. With recipes for every day of the week, it's easy to start to reduce the pain that chronic inflammation causes and reap the many benefits that this lifestyle choice has to offer. Let's take a look at what the anti-inflammatory diet is, what you can and can't eat, and what recipes will help you to get started in the right direction without sacrificing your taste buds.

WHAT IT IS

This is an eating plan that easily become a lifestyle, which is designed to both prevent and reduce chronic inflation. Chronic inflammation is a host to major diseases and health problems, which can all be avoided with the right dietary changes. The anti-inflammatory diet emphasizes whole foods such as vegetables, fruits, lean proteins, nuts, seeds and healthy fats. Chronic inflammation often comes from lifestyle factors including lack of exercise and high stress.

It is a result when your immune systems releases the chemicals to cause inflammation, thinking that it's combatting injury, virus infections or bacterial infections. Sadly, with chronic inflammation there is no real invaders for the body to fight off. Since food choices also influence the amount of inflammation in your body, the diet is a great way to treat and prevent many conditions, which we'll talk more about in the benefit section of this book.

Symptoms to Look For

Here are the symptoms of chronic inflammation that you should look out for.

- Depression
- Stomach Issues (Long Term)
- Inflamed or Irritable Bowel (Including Diarrhea, Pain When Evacuating & Cramping)
- Swelling, Redness, Loss of Function, Coldness in Parts of the Body
- Pain
- Breathing Problems

Foods to Eat

There are many studies that show people with a high intake of fish, healthy oils, nuts, fruits, seeds and vegetables have reduces risk for disease that are related to inflammation. These substances are found in many foods. Antioxidants and omega-3 fatty acids are great at providing an anti-inflammatory effect. Here is a list of foods that are high in antioxidants.

- Apples
- Artichokes
- Avocados
- Berries
- Cherries
- Dark Green Leafy Vegetables (Kale, Collard Greens, Spinach, Etc.)
- Sweet Potatoes
- Broccoli
- Nuts (Such as Almonds, Hazelnuts, Pecans, Walnuts, Etc.)
- Beans (Such as Pinto, Black, Red, Etc.)
- Whole Grains (Including Oats and Brown Rice)
- Dark Chocolate (At Least 70%)

Here is a list of foods that are rich in omega-3 Fatty Acids

- Oily Fish (Including Salmon, Mackerel, Anchovies, Sardines and Herring)
- Walnuts
- Omega-3 Fortified Foods (Including Milk & Eggs)
- Flaxseeds

Herbs & Spices to alleviate inflammation include:

- Ginger
- Turmeric
- Garlic

Foods to Avoid

You should avoid Omega-6 fatty acids since they are an essential fatty acids that's also found in food but it will increase inflammatory chemicals. They do help to maintain bone health, promote brain function and regulate your metabolism though, so you shouldn't cut them from your diet completely. It's important to balance your omega-3 fatty acids with your omega-6 fatty acids so that your inflammation stays in check. Here are some foods that are high in omega-6 fatty acids.

- Meat
- Dairy Products
- Vegetable Oils

- Margarine

Here is a list of bad foods that you should avoid.

- Fats & Fatty Proteins
- Fast Food
- Fried Foods
- Egg Rolls (Fried)
- Bacon
- Hot Dogs
- Margarine
- Vegetable Shortening
- Pork
- Red Meat
- Sausage
- Cold Cuts
- Whipped Spreads
- Jerky
- Pizza
- Premixed Spices
- Bagels
- Sugary Breakfast Cereal
- Bread
- Cornbread
- Cornstarch
- Croissants
- Crackers
- Doughnuts
- Granola
- Most Muffins
- Flour
- Noodles
- Waffles
- Pancakes
- Pita Bread
- White Rice

- Tortilla or Taco Shells
- Candy
- Cake
- Most Cookies
- Artificial Sweeteners
- Whole Milk
- Most Cheeses (Except Romano, Feta & Parmesan)
- Cottage Cheese
- Ice Cream
- Mayonnaise
- Sugar
- Fruit Juice
- Jams & Jellies
- Molasses
- Pastries
- Pudding
- Pie
- Soda
- Honey (Some Raw Honey is fine)
- Corn Syrup
- Coffee Drinks
- Rice Cakes
- Corn Chips
- Chips
- Peanuts
- Popcorns
- Pretzels

How to Get Started

Start by cleaning out your kitchen for anything you aren't supposed to be eating on the anti-inflammatory diet. Keep your kitchen clean from these foods for at least a few weeks. While you can enjoy other foods in moderation, it's important that you avoid temptation as much as possible when switching over. Take a few anti-inflammatory recipes from this book, and start a meal plan. Try to plan at least one week in ahead, and remember to utilize leftovers. Changing over to this new diet shouldn't be difficult, so streamline the process as much as possible.

When shopping, you'll want to shop the perimeter of the store to avoid processed foods as much as possible. Think about the lifestyle that you currently have, and work to fit your anti-inflammatory diet into that. If you try to change your lifestyle instead, you're going to be more likely to fail. If you're busy? Eat more salads for lunch since you can bring it with you. If you enjoy beef? Try to get leaner cuts of meat and only indulge once or twice a week.

TOP 15 FOODS

You now know the basics of what you should and shouldn't be eating on the anti-inflammatory diet, but let's take a deeper look into what your diet should concentrate on. Here are the top 15 foods to include into your anti-inflammatory diet and why.

Bell Peppers

Any bell pepper can help, but red bell pepper is best. They're a great source of both capsaicin and antioxidants, which are great at fighting inflammation. They're also versatile. There is quercetin in your bell pepper as well which will help your body to absorb the anti-inflammatory curcumin. However, if you are sensitive to nightshades then you should omit these from your diet.

Kale

Kale is a cruciferous vegetable which is high in antioxidants and fiber, making it great for salads. You can also cook with it, and it goes fantastic with garlic! It even makes great chips if you're looking for a quick snack.

Broccoli

Broccoli is immune boosting with the amount of antioxidants it has as well as vitamin C. it also is high in fiber, and it's a cruciferous vegetable. It's a great way to fight inflammation, and it acts as a complement to brown rice and lean cuts of beef. You can stir fry it too as an easy way to add it into your anti-inflammatory diet.

Spinach

As well as hosting antioxidants, spinach is full of vitamin C and K. it's a go-to ingredient because it's versatile. You can enjoy it sautéed or raw in salads. Throwing in a spinach and kale salad into your weekly routine will really help reduce chronic inflammation.

Blueberries

Blueberries are full of antioxidants, and you can add them to dessert or oatmeal. It's great in a smoothie too, making it easy to add them into your diet.

Tomatoes

Tomatoes are full of antioxidants, especially one called lycopene. However, if you are sensitive to nightshades, tomatoes are in the nightshade family and should be avoided as to not cause further inflammation. Garlic, basil and olive oil are a great pairing for tomatoes, and you can easily make them into a sauce to go over chicken or lentils.

Fatty Fish

We've already talked about omega-3 and omega-6 fatty acids, which fight inflammation. Omega-3 fatty acids fight inflammation when omega-6 fatty acids can raise it, and fish is a great way to help to combat this. Try to keep a one to one ration, but a two to one ration is also alright, with the omega-6 fatty acids being higher. However, the Western diet is high in mega-6 fatty acids, which can throw your body out of a natural routine. Many people' current ration can be as high as twenty-five to one, which means you're getting more omega-6 than you are omega-3, which is why so many people are recommended to take fish oil supplements. It'll help to keep the ratio from being so unbalanced. Fatty fish are what you should aim for when adding seafood into your anti-inflammatory diet. They go great with citrus fruits and greens!

Nuts

This is another great addition to any anti-inflammatory diet. Macadamias, cashews, walnuts, almonds and pecans are the best nuts for helping to reduce inflammation. You can sprinkle them onto vegetables, crush fish or chicken with them or just blend them into desserts or smoothies. They're high in calories, so you need to only stick to a handful a day if you are having weight issues.

Garlic

Garlic has been held in high regard for its anti-inflammatory properties, and it can boost your immune system too. It can also enhance flavors for lean meats, vinaigrettes, citrus sauces, plant based proteins, and stir fries. You can even use it to make hummus!

Cinnamon

This is another spice that can help to fight inflammation because it contains cinnamaldeyde, which inhibits inflammatory agents. It can be used for sweet and savory dishes, but the Western world mostly uses it for sweet dishes. You can use it for breakfast and dessert very easily.

Rosemary

Rosemary has a fantastic smell, so it brings an extra layer to your dish while still hosting anti-inflammatory benefits. It goes great on fish, chicken and lean meats.

You can even use it in a balsamic vinegar sauce or with strawberries to make a smoothie.

Ginger

Ginger is a powerful anti-inflammatory because it'll inhibit inflammation at a cellular level. It's an adaptive spice that will fit both sweet and savory foods, making it easy to use. Many people add it into soups, stir fries, or over dessert dishes with either apples or pears.

Turmeric

Turmeric has curcumin, which is great at fighting inflammation. However, if you're used to the traditional Wester diet, then you've probably not learned to incorporate turmeric into your cooking. You'll find a few turmeric recipes in this book to help you get started. It goes great in smoothies, curries, or on fish or poultry.

Olive Oil

Olive oil has a great fat profile because it contains oleocanthal which fights pro-inflammatory substances. Extra virgin olive oil is best, and you can use it to cook with or even toss on a salad, so it's easy to add into your diet.

Green Tea

Green tea is packed with antioxidants that support your immune system while fighting inflammation. You can drink it alone or you can add in some honey. Green tea powder, also known as matcha, can be added into fruit smoothies too.

More Foods to Enjoy

- Acorn squash
- Arugula
- Asparagus
- Artichoke
- Beet greens
- Beets
- Bok Choy
- Beans
- Brussel Sprouts
- Butternut Squash
- Carrots
- Cauliflower
- Cabbage
- Celeriac (Celery Root)
- Celery
- Collard Greens
- Chayote
- Cucumber
- Edamame
- Eggplant
- Endives
- Frisee
- Fennel
- Grape Leaves
- Hearts of Palms
- Jicama
- Kohlrabi Leeks
- Lettuce
- Mustard Greens
- Mushrooms
- Nori
- Nopales

- Okra
- Parsnip
- Onions
- Pattypan Squash
- Pea Pods
- Purslane
- Pumpkin
- Rutabaga
- Scallions
- Shallots
- Spinach
- Spaghetti Squash
- Sprouts
- Sweet potato
- Swiss chard
- Turnip
- Turnip Greens
- Water chestnuts
- Watercress
- Yam
- Zucchini

3 MAIN BENEFITS OF THIS DIET

You already know the main benefit of the anti-inflammatory diet, which is to reduce inflammation. However, that inflammation reduction does much more for your body than to just get rid of persistent discomfort and bloating. In this chapter, we'll explore the benefits of the anti-inflammatory diet.

Weight Loss

Wile you're also reducing your risk of developing chronic disease, one of the main benefits of this diet that attract people is weight loss. Without chronic inflammation, you'll find it easier to lose weight, especially when eating leaner cuts of meats and healthier food as a whole. With the anti-inflammatory diet, you have to say goodbye to the junk food, making it easier to get the vitamins and nutrients you need without the added calories.

Mood Booster

You have a lower risk of depression when you are getting the omega-3 Fatty acids that you need. Even if you're just added a fish oil supplement to your diet as well as fatty fish on occasion, you could experience a most increase. This is especially true for women.

Reduced Risk of Chronic Diseases

There are many diseases that are triggered by chronic inflammation. You'll find the list below.

- Many Cancers
- Cardiovascular disease
- Expression
- Diabetes
- Allergies
- Rheumatoid Arthritis
- Osteoporosis
- Obesity
- Pancreatitis
- Stroke
- Kidney Disease
- Respiratory Diseases
- Chhorn's Disease

- Alzheimer' Disease
- Macular Degeneration (Age Related)
- Irritable Bowel Syndrome
- Chronic Fatigue
- Fibromyalgia
- Celiac Disease
- Autoimmune Diseases

KITCHEN STAPLES

Here are some must have recipes that will be a staple to your anti-inflammatory diet.

Pistachio Pesto

Yields: 4 Cups
Serving: 4 Ounces
Calories: 229
Protein: 5.5 Grams
Fat: 3.6 Grams
Carbs: 3.8 Grams

Ingredients:

- 2 Cups Basil Leaves, Fresh & Packed Tight
- 1 Cup Pistachios, Raw
- ½ Cup Olive Oil, Divided
- ½ Cup Parmesan Cheese, Shredded
- 2 Teaspoon Lemon Juice, Fresh
- ½ Teaspoon Garlic Powder
- Sea Salt & Black Pepper to Taste

Directions:

1. Get out your food processor, and blend your basil, pistachios and a quarter cup of olive oil together for fifteen seconds.
2. Throw in your cheese, lemon juice, garlic powder, and then season with salt and pepper.
3. Pour in your remaining olive oil, and make sure it's mixed well. Serve immediately, and it will keep in the fridge for five days. You can also freeze it and it will keep for three months.

Caesar Dressing

Yields: ½ Cup
Serving: 2 Tablespoons
Calories: 167
Protein: 0.2 Grams
Fat: 18.9 Grams
Carbs: 1.3 Grams

Ingredients:

- ¼ Cup Paleo mayonnaise
- 2 Tablespoons Olive Oil
- 2 Cloves Garlic, Minced
- ½ Teaspoon Anchovy Paste
- 1 Tablespoon White Wine Vinegar
- ½ Teaspoon Lemon Zest
- 2 Tablespoons Lemon Juice, Fresh
- Sea Salt & Black Pepper to Taste

Directions:

1. Whisk all of your ingredients together. It should be emulsified and combined. Season with salt and pepper, and then refrigerate it for up to a week.

Beans

Serves: 5

Time: 1 Hour 5 Minutes

Calories: 153

Protein: 10 Grams

Fat: 1 Gram

Carbs: 28 Grams

Ingredients:

- 8 Ounces Beans, Dried
- Filtered Water (for Soaking & Cooking)
- 1 Bay leaf
- 1 Teaspoon Garlic
- 1 Teaspoon Onion Powder
- ½ Teaspoon Cumin
- Pinch Sea Salt, Fine

Directions:

1. Get out a glass bowl and add in your beans. Cover them with water, and then add a dash of salt. Let them soak for at least eight hours or overnight.

2. Drain them, and make sure to rinse well. Transfer them to a pot, and then season.

3. Cover with about two inches of water, and then cook on high heat. Bring it to a boil, and then reduce it to low. Allow it to simmer for an hour. Check to make sure your beans are done. If not, cook for ten minutes between checking until they're done.

Lemon Dijon Dressing

Serves: 13
Calories: 128
Protein: 0.1 Gram
Fat: 1.8 Grams
Carbs: 1.8 Grams

Ingredients:

- ¼ Cup Olive Oil
- 1 Teaspoon Dijon Mustard
- ½ Teaspoon Honey, Raw
- ¼ Teaspoon Basil
- 1 Clove Garlic, Minced
- ¼ Teaspoon Sea Salt, Fine
- 2 Tablespoons Lemon Juice, Fresh

Directions:

1.   Mix all ingredients together, and shake vigorously. Refrigerate for up to a week.

Tahini & Lime Dressing

Yields: ¾ Cup

Serving: 1 ½ Tablespoons

Time: 5 Minutes

Calories: 157

Protein: 6.2 Grams

Fat: 2.1 Grams

Carbs: 5.1 Grams

Ingredients:

- 3 Tablespoons Water
- 2 Tablespoons Lime Juice Fresh
- 1 Tablespoon Apple Cider Vinegar
- 1/3 Cup Tahini (Sesame Paste)
- 1 Teaspoon Lime Zest
- 1 ½ Teaspoons Honey, Raw
- Pinch Sea Salt, Fine
- ¼ Teaspoon Garlic Powder

Directions:

1.   Combine everything together, and shake vigorously until it I emulsified and combined. This will last in the fridge for up to a week.

Everything Aioli

Yields: ½ Cup
Serving: 2 Tablespoons
Calories: 43
Protein: 2 Grams
Fat: 2.4 Grams
Carbs: 3.2 Grams

Ingredients:

- ½ Cup Whole Milk
- 2 Teaspoons Dijon Mustard
- ¼ Teaspoon Honey, Raw
- ½ Teaspoon Hot Sauce
- Pinch Sea Salt

Directions:

1. Mix everything together, and it will keep in the fridge for up to three days.

Almond Romesco Sauce

Yields: 2 Cups
Time: 20 Minutes
Calories: 358
Protein: 7.3 Grams
Fat: 32.2 Grams
Carbs: 13.7 Grams

Ingredients:

- 2 Red Bell Peppers, Chopped Rough
- 6 Cherry Tomatoes, Chopped Rough
- 3 Cloves Garlic, Chopped Rough
- ½ White Onion, Chopped Rough
- 1 Tablespoon Avocado Oil
- 1 Cup Raw Almonds, Blanched
- ¼ Cup Olive Oil
- 2 Tablespoons Apple Cider Vinegar
- Sea Salt & Black Pepper to taste

Directions:

1. Turn your broiler to high and allow it to preheat. Get out a baking sheet and line it with foil.
2. Spread your tomatoes, onion, garlic and bell pepper onto your baking sheet, and drizzle it with avocado oil. Broil this for ten minutes, and then get out a blender.
3. Pulse your almonds until they are crumbly.
4. Add in your olive oil, vinegar, vegetables, salt and pepper. Process until smooth. It can keep in the fridge for up to five days. Alternatively, you can freeze it and it will keep for three months.

BREAKFAST RECIPES

Breakfast is an important meal of the day, and skipping it doesn't set you up for success. These recipes are easy and healthy.

Coconut Pancakes

Serves: 4
Time: 25 Minutes
Calories: 340
Protein: 10 Grams
Fat: 29 Grams
Carbs: 10 Grams

Ingredients:

- 1 Cup Coconut Milk, Unsweetened
- ¼ Teaspoon Sea Salt
- ½ Cup Coconut Flour
- ½ Teaspoon Baking Soda
- 4 Eggs, Lightly Beaten
- ½ Teaspoon Vanilla Extract, Pure
- 3 Tablespoons Olive Oil

Directions:

1. Whisk all of your ingredients together, and then melt a tablespoon of oil into a skillet using medium heat.
2. Add your batter in, and cook for two to three minutes per side. Use up all of your batter and serve warm.

Blueberry Matcha Smoothie

Serves: 2
Time: 5 Minutes
Calories: 208
Protein: 8.7 Grams
Fat: 5.7 Grams
Carbs: 31 Grams

Ingredients:

- 2 Cups Blueberries, Frozen
- 2 Cups Almond Milk
- 1 Banana
- 2 Tablespoons Protein Powder, Optional
- ¼ Teaspoon Ground Cinnamon
- 1 Tablespoon Chia Seeds
- 1 Tablespoon Matcha Powder
- ¼ Teaspoon Ground Ginger
- A Pinch Sea Salt

Directions:

1. Blend everything together until smooth.

Pumpkin Pie Smoothie

Serves: 2

Time: 5 Minutes

Calories: 235

Protein: 5.6 Grams

Fat: 11 Grams

Carbs: 27.8 Grams

Ingredients:

- 1 Banana
- ½ Cup Pumpkin, Canned & Unsweetened
- 2-3 Ice Cubes
- 1 Cup Almond Milk
- 2 Tablespoons Almond Butter, Heaping
- 1 Teaspoon Ground Nutmeg
- 1 Teaspoon Ground Cinnamon
- 1 Teaspoon Vanilla Extract Pure
- 1 Teaspoon Maple Syrup, Pure

Directions:

1. Blend everything together until smooth.

Leek & Spinach Frittata

Serves: 4

Time: 25 Minutes

Calories: 276

Protein: 19 Grams

Fat: 17 Grams

Carbs: 15 Grams

Ingredients:

- 2 Leeks, Chopped Fine
- 2 Tablespoons Avocado Oil
- 8 Eggs
- ½ Teaspoon Garlic Powder
- ½ Teaspoon Bail, Dried
- 1 Cup Baby Spinach, Fresh & Packed
- 1 Cup Cremini Mushrooms, Sliced
- Sea Salt & Black Pepper to Taste

Directions:

1. Start by heating your oven to 400, and then get out an ovenproof skillet. Place it over medium-high heat, sautéing your leeks in your avocado oil until soft. It should take roughly five minutes

2. Get out a bowl, and whisk the eggs with your garlic, basil, and salt. Add them to the skillet with your leeks, cooking for five minutes. You'll need to stir frequently.

3. Stir in your mushrooms and spinach, seasoning with pepper.

4. Place your skillet in the oven, baking for ten minutes. Serve warm.

Cherry Chia Oats

Serves: 2

Time: 30 Minutes

Calories: 564

Protein: 22 Grams

Fat: 32 Grams

Carbs: 27 Grams

Ingredients:

- ¼ Teaspoon Vanilla Extract, Pure
- 2 Tablespoons Almond Butter
- 8 Cherries, Fresh, Pitted & Halved
- 1 Cup Quick Cook Oats
- 2 Tablespoons Chia Seeds
- ¼ Cup Whole Milk Yogurt, Plain
- 1 ¼ Cup Almond Milk

Directions:

1. Stir all of your ingredients together until they're combined well.
2. Seal in two jars and refrigerate for twenty-five minutes before serving.

Banana Pancakes

Serves: 2

Time: 15 Minutes

Calories: 306

Protein: 15 Grams

Fat: 15 Grams

Carbs: 17 Grams

Ingredients:

- 2 Eggs
- 1 Egg White
- 1 Banana, Ripe
- 1 Cup Rolled Oats
- 2 Teaspoons Ground Cinnamon
- 1 Tablespoon Coconut Oil, Divided
- 1 Teaspoon Vanilla Extract, Pure
- ½ Teaspoon Sea Salt

Directions:

1. Get out a food processor, grinding your oats until they make a coarse flour.

2. Add your cinnamon, egg whites, eggs, banana, vanilla and salt. Blend until it forms a smooth batter, and then heat a small skillet over medium heat. Heat a half a tablespoon of coconut oil, and then pour your batter in. cook for two minutes per side, and continue until all of your batter has been used.

Turmeric Delight

Serves: 2

Time: 5 Minutes

Calories: 234

Protein: 9.3 Grams

Fat: 8.2 Grams

Carbs: 33.5 Grams

Ingredients:

- 2 Cups Yogurt, Plain & Whole Milk
- 1 Tablespoon Lemon Juice, Fresh
- 1 Banana, Sliced
- 2 Teaspoons Honey, Raw
- 1 Teaspoon Turmeric
- ½ Teaspoon Cinnamon
- ¼ Teaspoon Ginger

Directions:

1. Blend all of your ingredients together until smooth.

Fig Smoothie

Serves: 2

Time: 5 Minutes

Calories: 362

Protein: 9 Grams

Fat: 12 Grams

Carbs: 60 Grams

Ingredients:

- 7 Figs, Halved (Fresh or Frozen)
- 1 Banana
- 1 Cup Whole Milk Yogurt, Plain
- 1 Cup Almond Milk
- 1 Teaspoon Flaxseed, Ground
- 1 Tablespoon Almond Butter
- 1 Teaspoon Honey, Raw
- 3-4 Ice Cubes

Directions:

1. Blend everything together until smooth, and serve immediately.

LUNCH RECIPES

Lunch recipes vary depending on if you're on the go or able to stay at home. Usually, it's a mix of both, which is where this mixture comes in handy.

Open Avocado Tuna Melts

Serves: 4

Time: 15 Minutes

Calories: 471

Protein: 27 Grams

Fat: 27 Grams

Carbs: 31 Grams

Ingredients:

- 4 Slices Sourdough Bread
- 2 Cans Wild Caught Albacore Tuna, 5 Ounces
- ¼ Cup Paleo Mayonnaise
- 1 Teaspoon Lemon Juice, Fresh
- 2 Tablespoons Shallots, Minced
- Dash Garlic Powder
- Dash Paprika
- 1 Avocado, Cut into 8 Slices
- 1 Tomato, Cut into 8 Slices
- ¼ Cup Parmesan Cheese, Shredded & Divided

Directions:

1. Start by preheating your broiler, and then get out a baking sheet. Line it with foil.
2. Arrange your bread in the pan.
3. Get out a bowl, and then mix your mayonnaise, tuna, lemon juice, garlic, shallot and paprika together. Top each bread slice with the mixture.
4. Top each with two tomato slices and two avocado slices.
5. Sprinkle with a tablespoon of parmesan, and then broil for three to four minutes. Serve warm.

Carrot Salad

Serves: 6

Time: 10 Minutes

Calories: 101

Protein: 2 Grams

Fat: 2 Grams

Carbs: 22 Grams

Ingredients:

- ½ Cup Cilantro, Fresh & Chopped Fine
- 4 Carrots, Shredded
- 1/3 Cup Pistachios, Shelled & Roughly Chopped
- ¼ Teaspoon Red Pepper Flakes
- 3 Scallions, Sliced
- 4 Medjool Dates, Pitted & Chopped
- ½ Cup Tahini Lime Dressing

Directions:

1. Mix everything together and toss with your dressing before serving.

Chocolate Chili

Serves: 4
Time: 1 Hour
Calories: 370
Protein: 23 Grams
Fat: 27 Grams
Carbs: 9 Grams

Ingredients:

- 1 Tablespoon Olive Oil
- 1 Teaspoon Sea Salt
- 1 lb. Ground Beef, Lean
- 1 Onion, Large & Chopped
- 2 Cloves Garlic, Minced
- 1 ½ Teaspoons Chili Powder
- 1 Tablespoon Cocoa, Unsweetened
- ½ Teaspoon Ground Cumin
- 1 Cup Tomato Paste
- 2 Cups Chicken Broth

Directions:

1. Get out a Dutch oven, and then heat your oil over high heat.

2. Add in your ground beef, cooking until it browns. This should take about five minutes.

3. Add in your garlic, cocoa, chili powder, salt, cumin and onion. Allow it to cook for a minute more.

4. Add in your tomato sauce and chicken broth, bringing it to a simmer. Cover and cook for thirty to forty minutes. Make sure to stir occasionally. If it is too thick, add ore chicken broth to thin it.

5. Serve warm.

Mushroom Risotto

Serves: 4

Time: 25 Minutes

Calories: 320

Protein: 10 Grams

Fat: 11 Grams

Carbs: 829

Ingredients:

- 2 Tablespoons Olive Oil
- 1 Shallot, Large & Sliced Thin
- 10 Cremini Mushrooms, Sliced
- ½ Cup Red Wine, Dry
- 1 Cup Arborio Rice
- 1 ½ - 2 Cups Vegetable Broth
- ½ Cup Parmesan Cheese, Grated
- 1 Tablespoon Parsley, Freshly Chopped
- 1 Teaspoon Sea Salt, Fine
- Black Pepper to Taste

Directions:

1. Heat your oil in a skillet using high heat, and then add in your shallot. Cook for three to five minutes or until softened.

2. Add your mushrooms and red wine, simmering until the wine evaporates.

3. Add in your rice, cooking for three more minutes.

4. Add in a half a cup of your broth, cooking and stirring until it's been absorbed. Repeat until your risotto is tender, but it shouldn't be mushy. This should take roughly twenty minutes.

5. Remove from heat, sprinkling with parsley, parmesan, salt and pepper. Serve warm.

Mango & Avocado Salad

Serves: 2

Time: 10 Minutes

Calories: 500

Protein: 8 Grams

Fat: 39 Grams

Carbs: 40 Grams

Ingredients:

- 1 Romaine Lettuce Heart, Chopped
- ¼ Cup Dressing
- ¼ Cup Almonds, Toasted
- 1 Tablespoon Chives, Fresh & Chopped
- 1 Avocado, Peeled, Pitted & Sliced
- 1 Mango, Sliced

Directions:

1. Divide your lettuce between bowls, topping with mango and avocado.
2. Sprinkle with chives, and drizzle with salad dressing of your choice.
3. Top with almonds before serving.

Kale Salad

Serves: 6
Time: 30 Minutes
Calories: 213
Protein: 5 Grams
Fat: 14 Grams
Carbs: 22 Grams

Ingredients:

- 2 Tablespoons Apple Cider Vinegar
- 1 Teaspoon Sea Salt, Fine
- ½ Teaspoon Red Pepper Flakes
- ¼ Teaspoon Black Pepper
- 2 Sweet Potatoes Small & Peeled
- 1 Leek, Small
- 1 Apple, Peeled
- ¼ Cup Pine Nuts
- 1 Tablespoon Avocado Oil
- 3 Tablespoons Olive Oil
- 15 Ounces Kale, Stemmed & Chopped

Directions:

1. Start by heating your oven to 350.
2. Get out a baking sheet, and line it with parchment paper.
3. Combine your kale, olive oil, red pepper flakes, black pepper and vinegar. Knead these spices and oil into your kale for a minute. Transfer three quarters of this mixture to your baking pan, spreading it out. Bake for twenty minutes, tossing halfway through. Add it back to your remaining kale.
4. Chop your leeks, sweet potatoes, and apple into bite sized pieces, and then throw your avocado oil in a skillet. Place your skillet over medium heat, cooking the mixture for ten minutes. Your sweet potatoes should be soft.
5. Remove the kale from the oven, and then top your sweet potato mixture with it and pine nuts. Mix well before serving.

Spicy Ramen Soup

Serves: 4

Time: 15 Minutes

Calories: 663

Protein: 21 Grams

Fat: 28 Grams

Carbs: 115 Grams

Ingredients:

- 2 Tablespoons Sesame Seeds
- 8 Ounces Rice Noodles, Cooked
- ¼ Cup Cucumber, Sliced Thin
- ¼ Cup Scallion, Sliced
- ¼ Cup Cilantro, Fresh & chopped
- 2 Tablespoons Sesame Oil
- 1 Tablespoon Coconut Aminos
- 1 Tablespoon Ginger, Fresh, Grated & Peeled
- 2 Tablespoons Rice vinegar
- 1 Tablespoons Honey, Raw
- 1 Tablespoon Lime Juice, Fresh
- 1 Teaspoon Chili Powder

Directions:

1.   Mix your sesame seeds, cucumber, scallion, noodles, cilantro, sesame oil, ginger, coconut aminos, vinegar, honey, chili powder and lime juice together.

2.   Dive amount four soup bowls, and serve at room temperature.

Miso Soup with Greens

Serves: 4

Time: 15 Minutes

Calories: 44

Protein: 2 Grams

Fat: 0 Grams

Carbs: 8 Grams

Ingredients:

- 3 Cups Water
- 4 Scallions, Sliced Thin
- 3 Cups Vegetable Broth
- ½ Teaspoon Fish Sauce
- 1 Cup Mushrooms, Sliced
- 3 Tablespoons Miso Paste
- 1 Cup Baby Spinach, Fresh & Washed

Directions:

1. Get out a soup pot, placing it over high heat. Add in your fish sauce, water, broth, and mushrooms. Bring it to a boil before taking it off of heat.

2. Mix your miso paste and a half a cup of your broth together until the miso paste dissolves. Stir this mixture back into the soup.

3. Stir in your scallions and spinach, serving warm.

Chicken Chili

Serves: 4

Time: 30 Minutes

Calories: 304

Protein: 21 Grams

Fat: 4 Grams

Carbs: 46 Grams

Ingredients:

- 8 Ounce Can Green Chilies, Mild, Diced & With Liquid
- 4 Cups White Beans, Cooked & Drained
- 4 Cups Chicken Broth
- 4 Teaspoon Cumin, Ground
- 1 Teaspoon Chili Powder
- 2 Teaspoon Oregano, Dried
- 4 Cups Chicken, Shredded & Cooked
- ¼ Teaspoon Cayenne Pepper
- 2 Scallions, Sliced
- 1 Tablespoon Ghee
- 6 Cloves Garlic, Minced
- 2 Onions, Small & Chopped
- 1 Tablespoon Ghee

Directions:

1. Get out a soup pot, placing it over medium heat. Melt your ghee in it before adding your garlic and onion in. sauté for five minutes, stirring well.
2. Add in your chilies, cooking for another two minutes. Remember to stir.
3. Stir in your oregano, chili, cayenne, cumin, beans and broth. Bring the mixture to a simmer.
4. Add in your chicken, letting it come to a simmer again. Reduce the heat to medium-low, and cook for another ten minutes.
5. Top with scallions before serving warm.

Lentil Stew

Serves: 4

Time: 30 Minutes

Calories: 240

Protein: 10 Grams

Fat: 4 Grams

Carbs: 42 Grams

Ingredients:

- 1 Tablespoon Olive Oil
- 8 Brussels Sprouts, Halved
- 3 Carrots, Peeled & Sliced
- 1 Onion, Chopped
- 1 Turnip, Peeled, Quartered & Sliced
- 6 Cups Vegetable Broth
- 1 Clove Garlic, Sliced
- 15 Ounce Can Lentils, Drained & Rinsed
- 1 Cup Corn, Frozen
- 1 Tablespoon Parsley, Fresh & Chopped
- Sea Salt & Black Pepper to Taste

Directions:

1. Get out a Dutch oven and heat your oil over high heat, adding in your onion. Cook for three minutes. Your onions should soften.

2. Add in your carrots, turnip, garlic, and Brussels sprouts. Cook for three more minutes.

3. Throw in your broth, bringing it to a boil. Once it boils, reduce it to a simmer. Cook for five more minutes or until your vegetables are tender.

4. Add in your salt, pepper, parsley, corn and lentils. Cook enough for everything to heat all the way through, and serve warm.

SNACK RECIPES

No matter what diet you're on, you're likely to start snacking every once in a while. That's why it's so important to keep healthy snacks on hand.

Spiced Nuts

Serves: 2

Time: 25 Minutes

Calories: 180

Protein: 6 Grams

Fat: 16 Grams

Carbs: 7 Grams

Ingredients:

- ½ Cup Walnuts
- 1 Cup Almonds
- 1 Teaspoon Ground Turmeric
- ¼ Cup Sunflower Seeds
- ¼ Cup Pumpkin Puree
- ¼ Teaspoon Garlic Powder
- ½ Teaspoon Ground Cumin
- ¼ Teaspoon Red Pepper Flakes

Directions:

1. Start by heating the oven to 350.
2. Combine all ingredients together, and then get out a baking sheet. Spread your nuts over your baking sheet, cooking for ten to fifteen minutes.
3. Allow them to cool completely before you store them.

Easy Guacamole

Yields: 3 Cups
Serving: 3 Ounces
Time: 10 Minutes
Calories: 358
Protein: 7.3 Grams
Fat: 32.2 Grams
Carbs: 13.7 Grams

Ingredients:

- 4 Avocados, Halved & Pitted
- 1 Teaspoon Garlic Powder
- ½ Teaspoon Sea Salt

Directions:

1. Scoop your avocado flesh out, placing it in a bowl.

2. Add in your salt and garlic powder mashing until it's creamy. You can refrigerate it and it'll keep for two days.

Spicy Bean Dip

Yields: 3 ½ Cups
Serving: ½ Cup
Time: 10 Minutes
Calories: 166
Protein: 9.4 Grams
Fat: 0.6 Grams
Carbs: 34.2 Grams

Ingredients:

- 14 Ounce Can Black Beans, Drained & Rinsed
- 14 Ounce Can Kidney Beans, Drained & Rinsed
- 2 Cherry Tomatoes
- 2 Cloves Garlic
- 2 Tablespoons Water
- 1 Tablespoon Apple Cider Vinegar
- 2 Teaspoon Honey, Raw
- 1 Teaspoon Lime Juice, Fresh
- ¼ Teaspoon Sea Salt
- ¼ Teaspoon Ground Cumin
- Pinch Cayenne Pepper
- Black Pepper to Taste

Directions:

1. Combine all of your ingredients in a food processor, and blend until it's smooth. Cover, and refrigerate before serving. It can keep in the fridge for up to five days.

Cashew "Humus"

Yields: 1 Cup
Serving: 2 ½ Tablespoons
Time: 20 Minutes
Calories: 112
Protein: 2.9 Grams
Fat: 8.8 Grams
Carbs: 5.3 Grams

Ingredients:

- 1 Cup Cashews, Raw & Soaked in Water for 15 Minutes & Drained
- 2 Cloves Garlic
- ¼ Cup Water
- 1 Tablespoon Olive Oil
- 1 Teaspoon Lemon juice, Fresh
- 2 Teaspoon Coconut Aminos
- ½ Teaspoon Ground Ginger
- Pinch Cayenne Pepper
- ¼ Teaspoon Sea Salt, Fine

Directions:

1. Blend all ingredients together, and make sure to scrape the sides. Continue to blend until smooth, and then refrigerate it before serving. It will keep in the fridge for up to five days.

Roasted Garlic Chickpeas

Yields; 4 Cups

Serving: ¼ Cup

Time: 25 Minutes

Calories: 150

Protein: 6 Grams

Fat: 5 Grams

Carbs: 21 Grams

Ingredients:

- 4 Cups Cooked Chickpeas, Rinsed, Drained & Dried
- 1 Teaspoon Garlic Powder
- 1 Teaspoon Sea Salt
- Black Pepper to Taste
- 2 Tablespoons Olive Oil

Directions:

1. Start by heating your oven to 400.
2. Spread your chickpeas on a baking sheet, coating them with your olive oil.
3. Bake of twenty minutes, making sure to stir them at the ten-minute mark.
4. Place your hot chickpeas in a bowl, seasoning before sealing them in an airtight container. They'll keep at room temperature for up to two days.

Salt & Vinegar Kale Crisps

Yields: 2 Cups

Serving: 1 Cup

Time: 30 Minutes

Calories: 135

Protein: 1 Gram

Fat: 14 Grams

Carbs: 3 Grams

Ingredients:

- 4 Cups Kale, Torn into 2 Inch Pieces
- 2 Tablespoons Olive Oil
- 2 Tablespoon Apple Cider Vinegar
- 1 Teaspoon Sea Salt, Fine

Directions:

1. Start by heating your oven to 350. Get out a bowl, and combine all of your ingredients.

2. Place your kale on a baking sheet, baking for twenty to twenty-five minutes. Toss halfway through this time.

3. Store at room temperature in an airtight container. They'll keep for two days.

Sweet Potato Muffins

Serves: 12

Time: 40 Minutes

Calories: 143

Protein: 4 Grams

Fat: 7 Grams

Carbs: 12 Grams

Ingredients:

- 1 Cup Sweet Potato, Cooked & Pureed
- 1 ½ Cups Rolled Oats
- 1 Teaspoon Baking Powder
- ½ Teaspoon Baking Soda
- 1/3 Cup Coconut Sugar
- 1 Cup Almond Milk
- ¼ Cup Almond Butter
- 1 Egg
- 2 Tablespoons Olive Oil
- 1 Teaspoon Ground Cinnamon
- 1 Teaspoon Vanilla Extract, Pure
- ¼ Teaspoon Sea Salt

Directions:

1. Start by heating your oven to 375.

2. Line your muffin tin with liners, and then get out a food processor.

3. Pulse your oats until it forms a course flour. Transfer it to a small bowl before setting it to the side.

4. Add all of your ingredients except for the oat flour, blending until smooth.

5. Slowly add in your oat flour, pulsing until it's well incorporated.

6. Divide between your cupcake liners, and bake for twenty to twenty-five minutes. Allow them to cool for at least five minutes before serving.

DINNER RECIPES

In this chapter we'll explore main dishes as well as one stop dishes where you won't need any sides.

Crusted Cod with Fruity Salsa

Serves: 4
Time: 25 Minutes
Calories: 369
Protein: 18 Grams
Fat: 27 Grams
Carbs: 18 Grams

Ingredients:

Salsa:
- 1 Cup Mango, Diced
- 1 Cup Pineapple, Diced
- ½ Avocado, Diced
- 1 Lime, Juiced
- ¼ Teaspoon Sea Salt, Fine
- Dash Chili Powder

Cod:
- 2 Tablespoons Avocado Oil
- 1 Cup Coconut, Dried & Unsweetened
- 1 Egg
- 4 Cod Fillets, 4 Ounces Each
- ½ Teaspoon Garlic Powder
- ¼ Teaspoon Cayenne Pepper
- 1 Teaspoon Sea Salt, Fine

Directions:

1. Get out a bowl and stir all of your salsa ingredients together. Make sure it's mixed well.
2. Get out a shallow bowl and beat your eggs. Place the coconut in another shallow bowl.
3. Dip each cod fillet into egg, and then coat it with coconut. Place it on a plate.
4. Sprinkle each fillet with garlic, cayenne pepper and salt.
5. Heat up a skillet over medium-high heat, heating up your avocado oil.
6. Cook each fillet for four to five minutes. Make sure to flip one in between.
7. Serve warm and topped with salsa.

Spicy Trout & Spinach

Serves: 4

Time: 25 Minutes

Calories: 160

Protein: 19 Grams

Fat: 7 Grams

Carbs: 5 Grams

Ingredients:

- Olive Oil for Brushing
- ½ Red Onion, Sliced Thin
- 4 Trout Fillets, Boneless
- 10 Ounce Package Spinach, Frozen & Thawed
- 2 Tablespoons Lemon Juice, Fresh
- ¼ Teaspoon Garlic Powder
- ¼ Teaspoon Chipotle Powder
- 1 Teaspoon Sea Salt, Fine

Directions:

1. Start by heating your oven to 375, and then get out a nine by thirteen inch baking pan. Brush it down with olive oil, adding in your spinach and red onion. Lay your trout on top.

2. Sprinkle it with chipotle power, garlic and sprinkle with salt.

3. Cover with foil, baking for fifteen minutes.

4. Drizzle with lemon juice before serving.

Garlic & Mustard Steak

Serves: 4

Time: 1 Hour

Calories: 480

Protein: 48 Grams

Fat: 31 Grams

Carbs: 3 Grams

Ingredients:

- 2 Tablespoons Dijon Mustard
- ½ Cup Balsamic Vinegar
- ½ Cup Olive Oil
- 2 Cloves Garlic, Minced
- 1 Teaspoon Rosemary, Fresh & Chopped
- 4 Steaks, 6 Ounces Each & ½ Inch Thick
- Sea Salt & Black Pepper to Taste

Directions:

1. Whisk everything but your steak together to create the marinade. Add your steaks in so that they're well coated. Cover, and allow them to marinate for a half hour.

2. Heat a skillet over high heat, and then blot your steaks with a paper towel after removing the fro the marinade.

3. Cook them in the skillet and flip once. It should be two to three minutes per side. Allow your steak to rest for five minutes before serving.

Feta & Chickpea Casserole

Serves: 6

Time: 45 Minutes

Calories: 210

Protein: 10 Grams

Fat: 12 Grams

Carbs: 16 Grams

Ingredients:

- ½ Cup Feta Cheese, Crumbled
- 1 Teaspoon Oregano, Dried
- 15 Ounce Can Chickpeas, Drained & Rinsed
- 2 Cloves Garlic, Chopped
- 1 Zucchini, Chopped
- 2 Tablespoons Olive Oil + Extra
- 1 Onion, Large & Chopped
- ½ Teaspoon Ground Cumin
- 4 Eggs, Beaten Lightly
- Sea Salt & Black Pepper to Taste

Directions:

1.   Start by preheating your oven to 350, and then brush a nine by thirteen inch baking pan with olive oil.

2.   Get out a skillet, heating up two tablespoons of olive oil using high heat.

3.   Add in your garlic, onion and zucchini. Sauté until your vegetables have browned, which should take roughly five minutes. Transfer your vegetables to a bowl, adding in your chickpeas. Mash with a potato masher.

4.   Add in your remaining ingredients, and then spoon the mixture into the pan.

5.   Bake for twenty minutes, and allow it to cool before serving.

Easy Pork Loin

Serves: 4

Time: 1 Hour

Calories: 490

Protein: 76 Grams

Fat: 18 Grams

Carbs: 0 Grams

Ingredients:

- 1 Boneless Pork Loin, 3-4 lbs.
- 1 Cup Water
- 2 Tablespoons Olive Oil
- 1 Teaspoon Rosemary, Dried
- Sea Salt & Black Pepper to Taste

Directions:

1. Start by heating your oven to 375, and then pour your water into a nine by thirteen-inch pan.

2. Place a large skillet over high heat, and then brush your roast down with olive oil. Put it in the hot skillet, browning on all sides. It should take two to three minutes per side, and then place it in the roasting pan.

3. Season, and then cook for thirty to forty minutes.

4. Allow it to rest before serving.

Balsamic Chicken

Serves: 4

Time: 30 Minutes

Calories: 230

Protein: 35 Grams

Fat: 4 Grams

Carbs: 12 Grams

Ingredients:

- ¼ Cup Balsamic Vinegar
- 2 Tablespoons Honey, Raw
- 1 Teaspoon Sea Salt
- 1 Shallot, Minced
- 4 Chicken Breasts, Boneless & Skinless

Directions:

1. Start by heating your oven to 350.

2. Combine your shallot, salt, honey and vinegar together in a nine by thirteen-inch baking dish. Stir until the honey has dissolved. Add your chicken in, turning to coat.

3. Bake for twenty minutes, and allow it to rest for five minutes before serving.

Chickpea Curry

Serves: 4

Time: 30 Minutes

Calories: 422

Protein: 11 Grams

Fat: 18 Grams

Carbs: 55 Grams

Ingredients:

- 2 White Onions, Small & Diced
- 2 Cloves Garlic, Minced
- 2 Tablespoons Avocado Oil
- ½ Cup Vegetable Broth
- 1 Red Bell Pepper, Chopped
- ½ Cup Cashews, Chopped Rough
- ½ Cup Golden Raisins
- 1 Apple, Diced
- ½ Teaspoon Sea Salt, Fine
- 1 Tablespoon Curry Powder
- 2 Cups Chickpeas, Cooked, Rinsed & Drained
- ½ Cup Whole Milk Yogurt, Plain

Directions:

1. Get out a large skillet, placing it over medium heat. Sauté your garlic and onion in avocado oil, cooking for two to three minutes.

2. Add in your bell pepper, and sauté for five minutes.

3. Stir in your salt, curry powder and broth. Bring it to a simmer.

4. Add your raisins, apple, and chickpeas. Cook for five minutes.

5. Stir in your cashews right before you turn off the heat, and then serve warm topped with yogurt.

Lentil Sloppy Joes

Serves: 4

Time: 30 Minutes

Calories: 277

Protein: 14 Grams

Fat: 7 Grams

Carbs: 29 Grams

Ingredients:

- 2 Tablespoons Avocado Oil, Divided
- 1 White Onion, Small & Chopped
- 1 Celery Stalk, Chopped Fine
- 1 Carrot, Minced
- 2 Cloves Garlic, Minced
- ½ Red Bell Pepper, Chopped Fine
- 1 lb. Lentils, Cooked
- 7 Tablespoons Tomato Paste
- 2 Tablespoons Apple Cider Vinegar
- 1 Tablespoon Maple Syrup, Pure
- 1 Teaspoon Chili Powder
- 1 Teaspoon Dijon Mustard
- ½ Teaspoon Oregano, Dried

Directions:

1.   Place a large pan over medium-high heat, adding gin a tablespoon of your avocado oil.

2.   Once your oil is hot, add in your garlic, carrot, onion and celery. Sauté for three minutes. Your onion should be translucent and tender.

3.   Add your lentils in with your remaining avocado oil, sautéing for another five minutes.

4.   Add in your red bell pepper, cooking for another two minutes.

5.   Stir in your remaining ingredients, cooking on medium-low for ten minutes. Serve over rice if desired.

Honey Garlic Scallops

Serves: 4
Time: 25 Minutes
Calories: 383
Protein: 21 Grams
Fat: 19 Grams
Carbs: 26 Grams

Ingredients:

- 1 lb. Scallops, Large & Rinsed
- Sea Salt & Black Pepper to Taste
- 2 Tablespoons Avocado Oil
- 3 Tablespoons Coconut Aminos
- ¼ Cup Honey, Raw
- 1 Tablespoon Apple Cider Vinegar
- 2 Cloves Garlic, Minced

Directions:

1. Use a paper towel to pat your scallops dry, seasoning them with salt and pepper.
2. Get out a skillet, placing it over medium-high heat, heating up your avocado oil.
3. Place your scallops in the skillet, cooking for two to three minutes per side. They should be golden. Transfer them to a plate, and place foil over them loosely to keep them warm. Tent the foil so that your scallops don't sweat.
4. In the same skillet, stir in your remaining ingredients, bringing it to a simmer. Cook for even minutes, and make sure to stir while the liquid reduces.
5. Return your scallops to your pan to glaze them, serving warm.

Miso Salmon

Serves: 4

Time: 15 Minutes

Calories: 264

Protein: 30 Grams

Fat: 9 Grams

Carbs: 13 Grams

Ingredients:

- 4 Salmon Fillets, 4 Ounces Each
- 3 Tablespoons Miso Paste
- 2 Tablespoons Honey, Raw
- 1 Teaspoon Coconut Aminos
- 1 Teaspoon Rice Vinegar

Directions:

1. Heat your broiler, and then get out a baking dish. Line it with foil, and place your salmon fillets in it.

2. Get out a bowl, stirring all of your ingredients together, and brush this glaze over the salmon.

3. Broil for five minutes, and brush down with the remaining glaze. Broil for another five minutes if needed.

Stuffed Bell Pepper

Serves: 6
Time: 30 Minutes
Calories: 188
Protein: 15 Grams
Carbs: 11 Grams

Ingredients:

- 6 Bell Peppers, Tops Removed & Deseeded
- 1 Tablespoon Avocado Oil
- 1 lb. Ground Turkey
- 1 Onion, Small & Diced
- 2 Cloves Garlic, Minced
- 16 Ounce Can Tomatoes, Drained
- ½ Teaspoon Paprika
- ½ Teaspoon Ground Cumin
- ½ Teaspoon Oregano, Dried
- Sea Salt & Black Pepper to Taste

Directions:

1. Start by heating your oven to 400, and then line a baking sheet with foil.
2. Arrange your bell peppers on it, drizzling them with your oil.
3. Bake for twenty minutes. They should be cooked and softened.
4. During this time get out a skillet, placing it over medium-high heat. Brown your turkey and break up any clumps. This should take roughly five minutes, and then add in your garlic and onion. Cook for twenty minutes while stirring frequently. Your turkey should be cooked all the way through.
5. Stir in your remaining ingredients, scooping this mixture into your bell pepper. Serve warm.

SIDE DISH RECIPES

For the main dishes you fell in love with, try to pair them with a side dish from this chapter to stick to your diet.

Arugula & Quinoa Tabbouleh

Serves: 6

Time: 10 Minutes

Calories: 235

Protein: 5 Grams

Fat: 14 Grams

Carbs: 24 Grams

Ingredients:

- ½ Cup Flat Leaf Parsley, Fresh & Chopped
- 3 Cups Quinoa, Cooked
- 1 Cup Arugulas, Packed
- 4 Scallions, Sliced
- ½ Cup Tomato, Diced
- ½ Cup Mint Leaves, Fresh & Minced
- 1/3 Cup Olive Oil
- ½ Teaspoon Garlic Powder
- ½ Teaspoon Sea Salt, Fine
- Black Pepper to Taste
- 2 Tablespoons Lemon Juice, Fresh

Directions:

1. Mix together your tomato, parsley, mint, scallions, arugula and quinoa.
2. In a bowl whisk together your lemon juice, garlic, salt, pepper and olive oil.
3. Toss your salad in the dressing before serving.

Wild Rice Salad

Serves: 8
Time: 25 Minutes
Calories: 143
Protein: 5 Grams
Fat: 4 Grams
Carbs: 22 Grams

Ingredients:

- 3 Cups Wild Rice, Cooked
- 2 Tablespoons Ghee
- 3 Cloves Garlic, Minced
- 1 Sweet Onion, Small & Diced
- 2 Cups Cremini Mushrooms, Sliced
- ½ Teaspoon Thyme, Dried
- ½ Cup Vegetable Broth
- ½ Teaspoon Sea Salt, Fine

Directions:

1. Place your rice in a bowl before setting it to the side.

2. Get out a saucepan, placing it over medium heat. Melt your ghee before adding in your garlic and onion. Cook for five minutes, and make sure to stir frequently.

3. Stir in your broth, thyme, salt and mushrooms. Allow it to cook for even to ten minutes. Your mushrooms should be tender, and the broth should reduce by half.

4. Add in the rice and mushroom mixture. Stir well, and serve warm.

Sweet Korean Lentils

Serves: 4
Time: 30 Minutes
Calories: 281
Protein: 14 Grams
Fat: 5 Grams
Carbs: 45 Grams

Ingredients:

- 1 Tablespoon Avocado Oil
- 1 White Onion, Small & Diced
- 2 Cloves Garlic, Minced
- 2 Cups Vegetable Broth
- 1 Cup Lentils, Dried, Sorted & Rinsed
- 3 Tablespoons Coconut Aminos
- 1 Teaspoon Sesame Oil
- 1 Tablespoon Rice Vinegar
- ¼ Teaspoon Red Pepper Flakes
- ½ Teaspoon Ginger, Ground
- 1 Tablespoon Sesame Seeds
- 2 Scallions, Sliced

Directions:

1.   Get out a stockpot, placing it over medium heat before adding in your avocado oil, garlic and onion. Sauté, cooking for five minutes. The onion should be translucent.

2.   Add in your lentils, coconut aminos, broth, vinegar, sesame oil, ginger, coconut sugar, ginger, and red pepper flakes.

3.   Increase your heat to medium-high, bringing it to a simmer. Reduce your heat to low, and then cover. Allow it to cook for fifteen minutes. The lentils should be cooked. Garnish with scallions and sesame seeds.

Citrus Spinach

Serves: 4
Time: 20 Minutes
Calories: 80
Protein: 1 Gram
Fat: 7 Grams
Carbs: 4 Grams

Ingredients:

- 2 Tablespoons Olive Oil
- 2 Cloves Garlic, Minced
- 4 Cups Baby Spinach, Fresh
- ½ Orange, Juiced & Zested
- ½ Teaspoon Sea Salt
- 1/8 Teaspoon Black Pepper

Directions:

1. Get out a large skillet, placing it over medium-high heat. Heat you olive oil until it begins to shimmer.

2. Add in your spinach, and cook for three minutes. Make sure to stir occasionally.

3. Add in your garlic, cooking for another thirty seconds. You'll need to stir constantly.

4. Add in your orange zest, orange juice, salt and pepper, cooking for two more minutes. Stir constantly until your juice evaporates, and then serve warm.

Brown Rice & Bell Pepper

Serves: 4

Time: 20 Minutes

Calories: 266

Protein: 5 Grams

Fat: 8 Grams

Carbs: 44 Grams

Ingredients:

- 2 Cups Brown Rice, Cooked
- 2 Tablespoon Soy Sauce, Low Sodium
- 2 Tablespoons Olive Oil
- 1 Red Bell Pepper, Chopped
- 1 Green Bell Pepper, Chopped
- 1 Onion, Chopped

Directions:

1. Get out a nonstick skillet, placing it over medium-high heat. Add in your olive oil, heating it up until it shimmers.

2. Add in your onion and bell pepper, cooking for seven minutes. Make sure to stir frequently. The vegetable should brown.

3. Add in your soy sauce and rice, cooking or three minutes. Stir constantly. Your rice should be warmed.

Green Pasta Salad

Serves: 4

Time: 30 Minutes

Calories: 450

Protein: 13 Grams

Fat: 15 Grams

Carbs: 68 Grams

Ingredients:

- 2 Cups Arugula
- 1 Cup Basil Sauce
- 1 Tablespoon Olive Oil
- 1 Bunch Asparagus, Sliced into 1 Inch Pieces
- 12 Ounces Penne
- 2 Scallions, Sliced
- Sea Salt & Black Pepper to Taste

Directions:

1. Start by cooking your pasta per package instructions, and add in your asparagus for the last two minutes.

2. Drain this mixture using a colander before putting them back in the pot.

3. Add in your sauce and oil, stirring until it's combined.

4. Allow it to cool to room temperature, and then stir in your remaining ingredients. Serve warm.

Roasted Potatoes

Serves: 4

Time: 25 Minutes

Calories: 180

Protein: 3 Grams

Fat: 7 Grams

Carbs: 27 Grams

Ingredients:

- 2 Tablespoons Olive Oil
- 1 ½ lbs. Fingerling Potatoes, Scrubbed
- 1 Teaspoon Sea Salt, Fine
- ¼ Teaspoon Black Pepper
- 1 Tablespoon Parsley, Fresh & Chopped

Directions:

1. Start by heating your oven to 400, and then get out a baking sheet. Brush it with oil, and place your potatoes in a bowl. Toss with two tablespoons of oil. It should be coated. Season with salt and pepper, and arrange on a baking sheet in a single layer.

2. Bake for twenty minutes. They should be tender and browned lightly. Sprinkle with parsley before serving.

Rosemary Rice

Serves: 4

Time: 55 Minutes

Calories: 190

Protein: 6 Grams

Fat: 4 Grams

Carbs: 33 Grams

Ingredients:

- 1 Cup Wild Rice
- 3 ½ Cups Vegetable Broth
- 1 Teaspoon Sea Salt, Fine
- 1 Tablespoon Olive Oil
- ¼ Teaspoon Black Pepper
- 1 Teaspoon Rosemary, Fresh & Chopped

Directions:

1. Rinse your rice using a fine mesh strainer, and drain well. Place it in a pot, adding in your broth, salt, pepper and olive oil.

2. Bring it to a boil using high heat before reducing it to simmer. Cover the pot partially so that steam escapes. Allow it to cook for thirty-five to forty-five minutes.

3. Drain any remaining liquid, adding your rosemary, and fluff before serving.

Broccoli Slaw

Serves: 4

Time: 10 Minutes

Calories: 110

Protein: 2 Grams

Fat: 7 Grams

Carbs: 12 rams

Ingredients:

- ¼ Cup Cranberries, Dried
- ¼ Cup Almonds, Sliced
- 2 Scallions, Sliced
- 1 Head Broccoli, Chopped into Bite Size Pieces
- 1 Tablespoon Paleo Mayonnaise
- 2 Tablespoons Whole Milk Yogurt, Plain
- 1 Tablespoon Lemon Juice, Fresh
- 1 Teaspoon Honey, Raw
- ½ Teaspoon Ground Cumin
- Dash Hot Sauce
- Sea Salt & Black Pepper to Taste

Directions:

1. Combine your scallions, cranberries, almonds and broccoli together.

2. Get out a different bowl and whisk your remaining ingredients together to make your dressing. Pour this over your broccoli mixture, and mix well before serving.

Sautéed Bok Choy

Serves: 4

Time: 20 Minutes

Calories: 143

Protein: 12 Grams

Fat: 5 Grams

Carbs: 21 Grams

Ingredients:

- 2 Tablespoons Coconut Aminos
- 1 Tablespoon Sesame Oil
- 1 Teaspoon Ginger, Peeled & Minced
- 2 Cloves Garlic, Minced
- 3 Tablespoons Water
- 1 Teaspoon Rice Vinegar
- ¼ Teaspoon Red Pepper Flakes
- 4 Heads Bok Choy, Halved Lengthwise

Directions:

1. Get out a large saucepan, placing it over medium heat. Warm your sesame oil before adding in your garlic and ginger. Cook for two minutes.

2. Stir in your vinegar, coconut aminos, red pepper flakes and water before adding your bok choy. Make sure that the cut sides are placed down, and then lower the heat to low. Cover your pan, allowing them to steam for five to ten minutes. They should be tender. Serve warm.

Mixed Beet Salad

Serves: 6

Time: 5 Minutes

Calories: 107

Protein: 4 Grams

Fat: 4 Grams

Carbs: 15 Grams

Ingredients:

- 6 Cups Mixed Greens
- 1 Cup English Peas, Shelled, Frozen & Thawed
- 3 Small Chioggia Beets, Sliced Thin
- 1 Red Onion, Small & Sliced
- 1 Avocado, Sliced
- ¼ Cup Lemon Dijon Mustard Dressing

Directions:

1. Mix everything together and then toss with the dressing before serving.

Root Mash

Serves: 4

Time: 30 Minutes

Calories: 270

Protein: 2 Grams

Fat: 10 Grams

Carbs: 23 Grams

Ingredients:

- 2 Cups Sweet Potatoes, Chopped
- 2 Cups Celery Root, Chopped, Trimmed & Peeled
- 1 Teaspoon Lemon Juice, fresh
- 2 Tablespoons Ghee
- ½ Teaspoon Sea Salt, Fine
- Pinch Cayenne Pepper

Directions:

1.   Get a steamer basket, placing it over boiling water. Place your celery root and sweet potatoes in it, steaming for twenty-five minutes using medium heat. They should be tender.

2.   Place them in a food processor, blending until smooth and then add in your remaining ingredients. Pulse until well combined, and serve warm.

Citrus Roasted Cauliflower

Serves: 4

Time: 25 Minutes

Calories: 138

Protein: 3 Grams

Fat: 11 Grams

Carbs: 9 Grams

Ingredients:

- 1 ½ Teaspoons Ground Cumin
- 1 Teaspoon Sea Salt, Fine
- ½ Teaspoon Chili Powder
- ½ Teaspoon Black Pepper
- 1 Head Cauliflower, Chopped Into Bite Size pieces
- ½ Teaspoon Garlic Powder
- 3 Tablespoons Ghee, Melted
- 3 Tablespoons Lime Juice, Fresh

Directions:

1. Start by heating your oven to 450.
2. Get out a bowl and mix your garlic, cumin, chili powder, salt and pepper.
3. Spread your cauliflower out evenly in a baking pan, drizzling with ghee and lime juice, sprinkling it with the spice mixture. Toss to make sure it's coated.
4. Bake for fifteen minutes.

Roasted Vegetables

Serves: 4
Time: 30 Minutes
Calories: 184
Protein: 2 Grams
Fat: 14 Grams
Carbs: 15 Grams

Ingredients:

- 2 Zucchini, Diced into 1 Inch Pieces
- 1 Red Bell Pepper, Diced into 1 Inch Pieces
- 1 Red Onion, Diced into 1 Inch Pieces
- 1 Yellow Bell Pepper, Diced into 1 Inch pieces
- 1 Sweet Potato, Diced into 1 Inch Pieces
- 4 Cloves Garlic
- ¼ Cup Olive Oil
- 1 Teaspoon Sea Salt, Fine

Directions:

1. Start by heating your oven to 450.
2. Line your baking sheet with foil, and then get out a bowl.
3. Toss your bell pepper, onion, zucchini, sweet potato, olive oil, salt and garlic. Spread this mixture out evenly on the baking sheet.
4. Bake for twenty-five minutes, stirring halfway through.

DESSERT RECIPES

No diet would be complete without at least a few dessert recipes that you can have, so try these delicious ones!

Avocado Fudge

Serves: 16

Time: 3 Hours 15 Minutes

Calories: 120

Protein: 1 Gram

Fat: 9 Grams

Carbs: 11 Grams

Ingredients:

- 1 Avocado, Peeled & Pitted
- ½ Teaspoon Sea Salt
- ¼ Cup Coconut Oil
- 1 ½ Cup Chocolate Chips, Bittersweet

Directions:

1.   Get out an eight-inch square baking pan, and then line it with parchment paper. Get out a double boiler, and melt your coconut oil and chocolate together.

2.   Transfer it to a food processor, allowing it to cool a little before adding in your avocado. Process until it is smooth.

3.   Spread this mixture into your pan, sprinkling with sea salt.

4.   Place it in the fridge for three hours before cutting it into sixteen pieces.

Caramelized Pears

Serves: 4
Time: 25 Minutes
Calories: 290
Protein: 12 Grams
Fat: 11 Grams
Carbs: 41 Grams

Ingredients:

- 1 Teaspoon Cinnamon
- 2 Tablespoon Honey, Raw
- 1 Tablespoon Coconut Oil
- 4 Pears, Peeled, Cored & Quartered
- 2 Cups Yogurt, Plain
- ¼ Cup Toasted Pecans, Chopped
- 1/8 Teaspoon Sea Salt

Directions:

1.	Get out a large skillet, and then heat the oil over medium-high heat.

2.	Add in your honey, cinnamon, pears and salt. Cover, and allow it to cook for four to five minutes. Stir occasionally, and your fruit should be tender.

3.	Uncover it, and allow the sauce to simmer until it thickens. This will take several minutes.

4.	Soon your yogurt into four dessert bowls. Top with pears and pecans before serving.

Berry Ice Pops

Serves: 4

Time: 3 Hours 5 Minutes

Calories: 140

Protein: 5 Grams

Fat: 4 Grams

Carbs: 23 Grams

Ingredients:

- 1 Cup Strawberries, Fresh or Frozen
- 2 Cups Whole Milk Yogurt, Plain
- 1 Cup Blueberries, Fresh or Frozen
- ¼ Cup Water
- 1 Teaspoon Lemon Juice, Fresh
- 2 Tablespoons Honey, Raw

Directions:

1. Place all of your ingredients in a blender, and blend until smooth.
2. Pour into your molds, and freeze for at least three hours before serving.

Fruit Cobbler

Serves: 8

Time: 30 Minutes

Calories: 196

Protein: 4 Grams

Fat: 12 Grams

Carbs: 15 Grams

Ingredients:

- 1 Teaspoon Coconut Oil
- ¼ Cup Coconut Oil, Melted
- 2 Cups Peaches, Fresh & Sliced
- 2 Cups Nectarines, Fresh & Sliced
- 2 Tablespoons Lemon Juice, Fresh
- ¾ Cup Rolled Oats
- ¾ Cup Almond Flour
- ¼ Cup Coconut Sugar
- ½ Teaspoon Vanilla Extract, Pure
- 1 Teaspoon Ground Cinnamon
- Dash Salt
- Filter Water for Mixing

Directions:

1. Start by heating your oven to 425.
2. Get out a cast iron skillet, coating it with a teaspoon of coconut oil.
3. Mix your lemon juice, peaches and nectarines together in the skillet.
4. Get out a food processor, mixing your almond flour, oats, coconut sugar, and remaining coconut oil. Add in your cinnamon, vanilla and salt, pulsing until the oat mixture resembles a dry dough.
5. If you need more moisture, add filtered water a tablespoon at a time, and then break the dough into chunks, spreading it across the fruit.
6. Bake for twenty minutes before serving warm.

Chocolate Cookies

Serves: 12
Time: 20 Minutes
Calories: 226
Protein: 6 Grams
Fat: 15 Grams
Carbs: 20 Grams

Ingredients:

- ¾ Cup Almond Butter, Creamy
- ½ Cup Coconut Sugar
- ¼ Cup Cocoa Powder
- 1 Egg
- 1 Egg Yolk
- 2 Teaspoons Vanilla Extract, Pure
- ½ Cup Chocolate Chips, Semi Sweet
- 1 Teaspoon Baking Soda
- ¼ Teaspoon Salt
- Dash Sea Salt

Directions:

1.   Start by preheating your oven to 350, and then get out a baking sheet. Line it with parchment paper, and get out a bowl cream your almond butter, cocoa powder, vanilla and coconut sugar together.

2.   Get out another bowl, whisking your egg and egg yolk together. Add this to your almond butter mixture. Stir to combine.

3.   Stir in your baking soda, salt and chocolate chips.

4.   Make twelve pieces, and roll them into balls. Place six per pan, and bake for nine to ten minutes.

5.   Allow them to rest for five minutes before sprinkling with sea salt, and serve cooled.

APPENDIX : RECIPES INDEX